BABY SHOWER

_____

_____

_____

_____

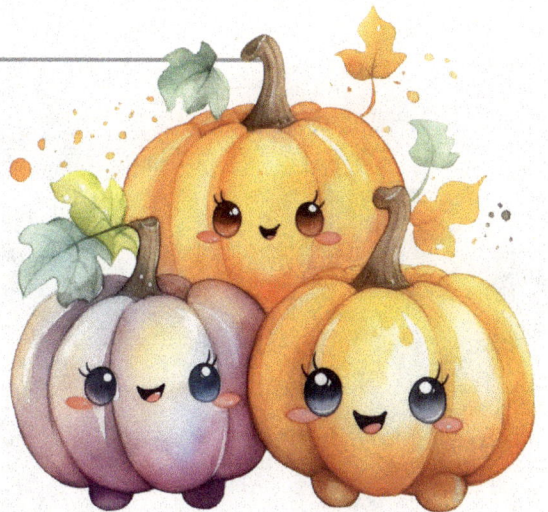

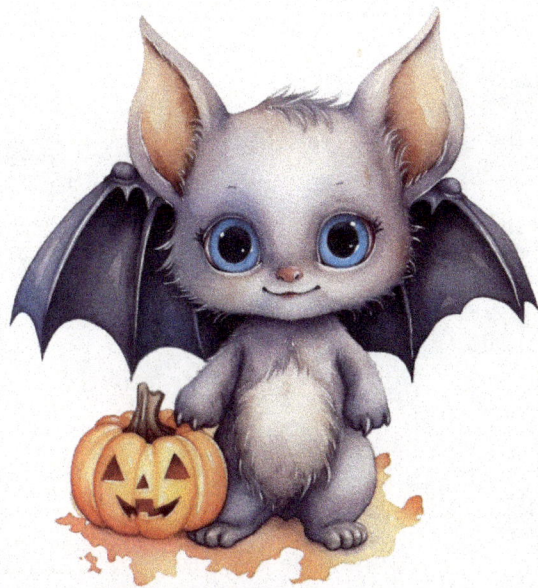

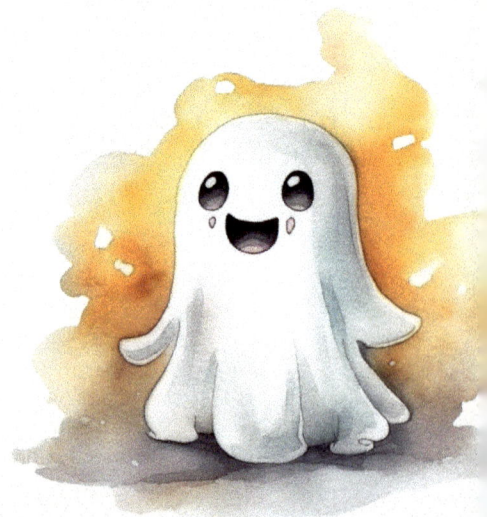

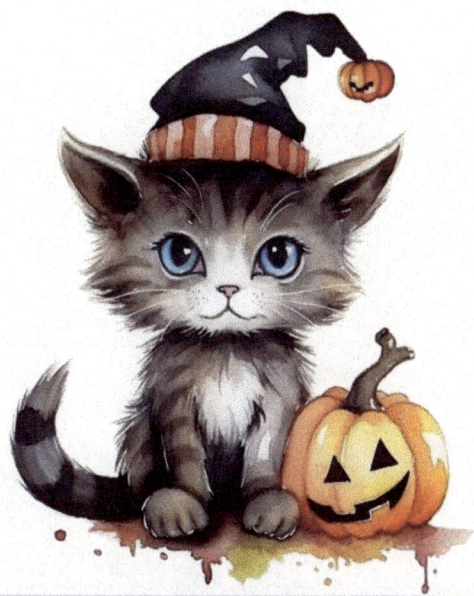

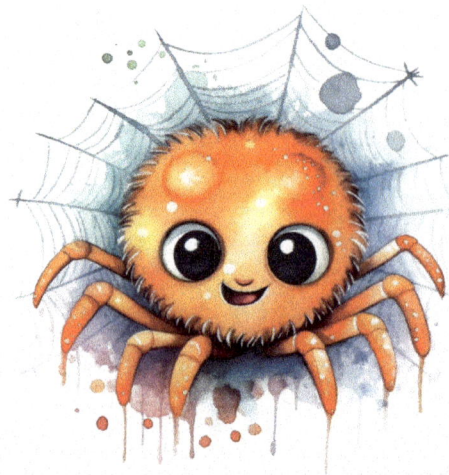

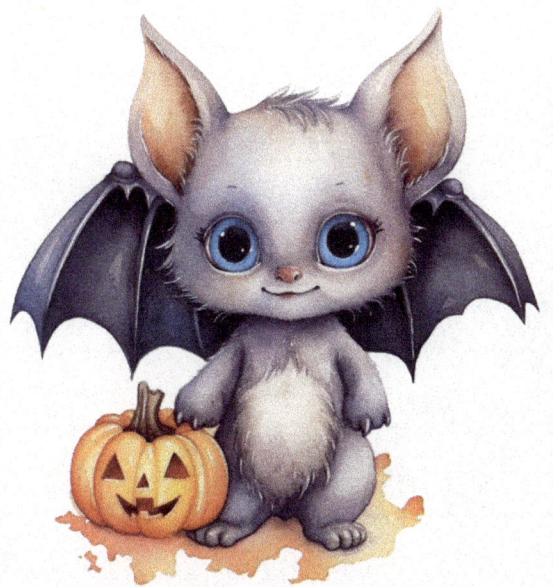

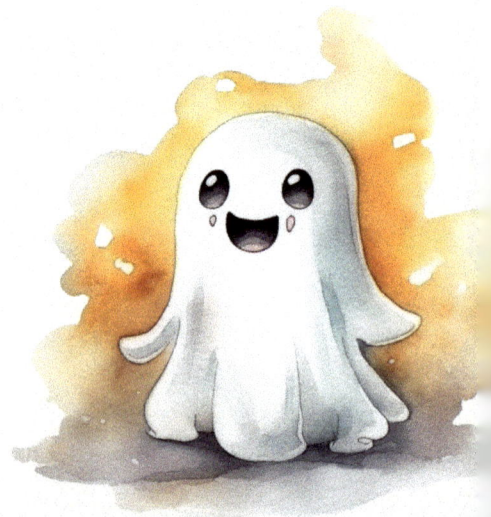

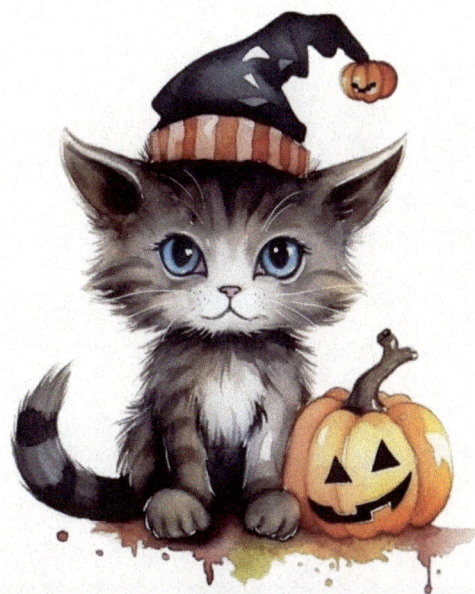

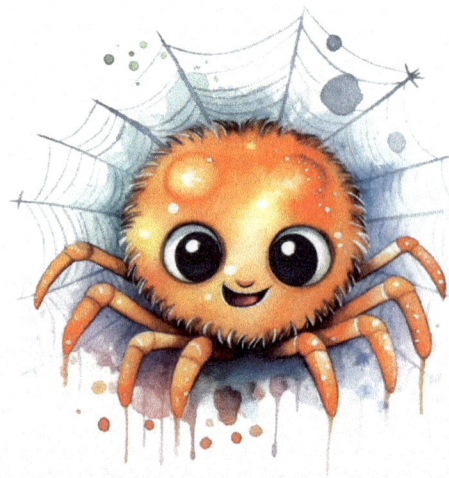

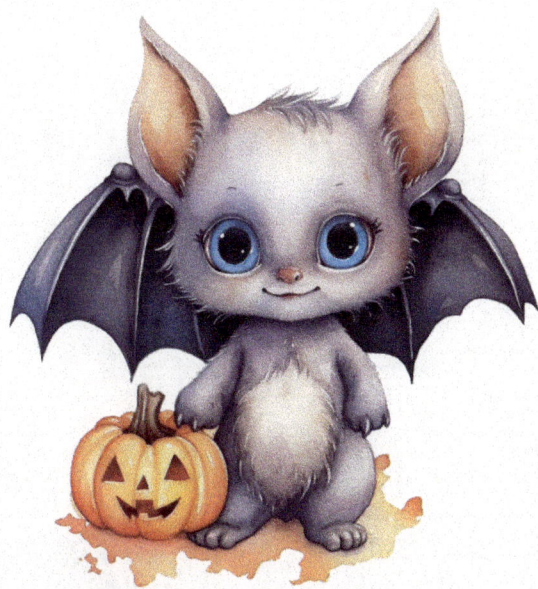

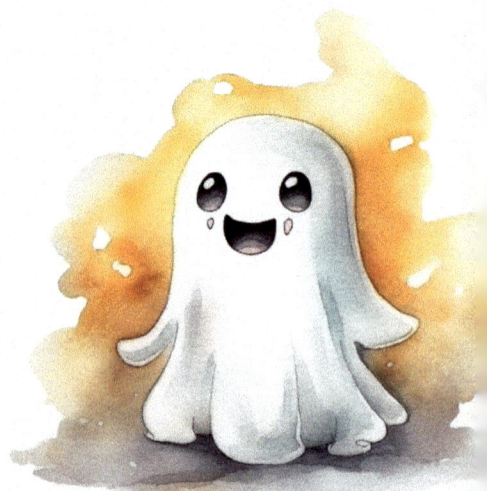

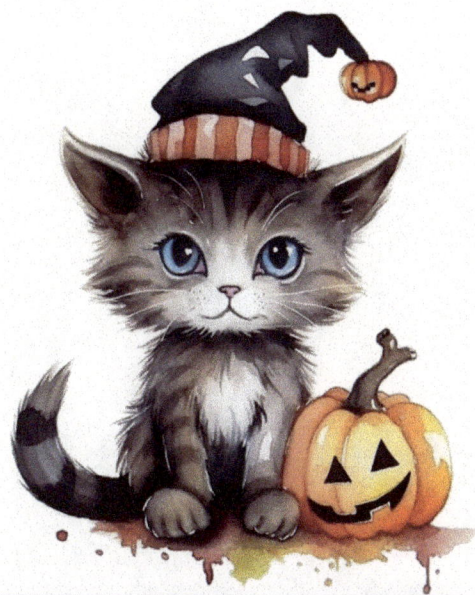

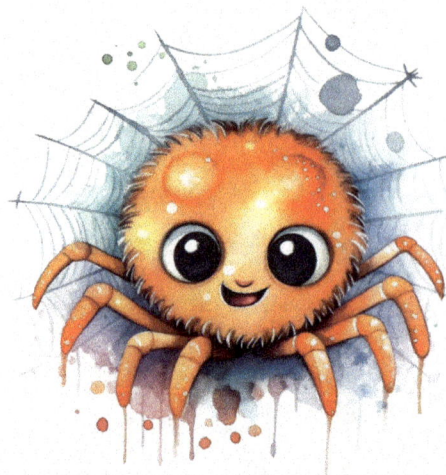

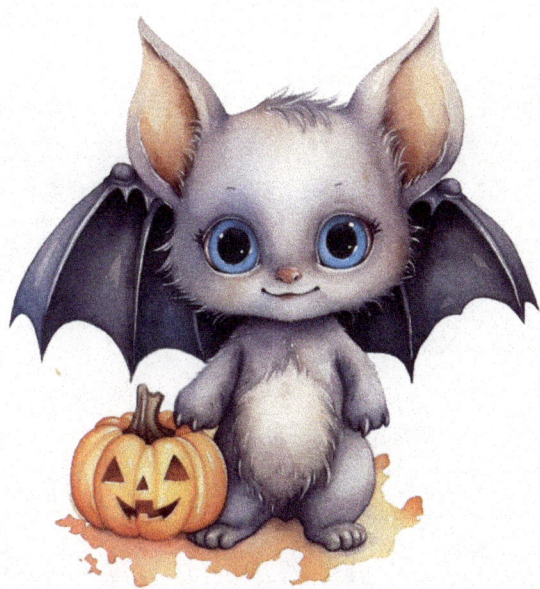

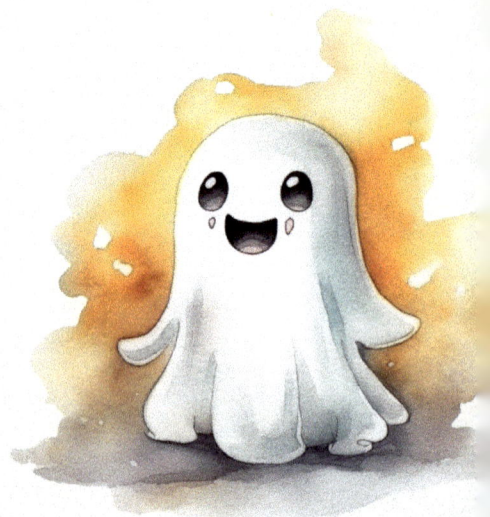

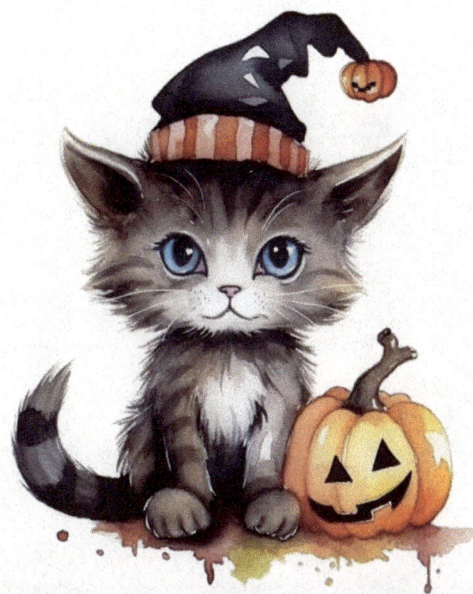

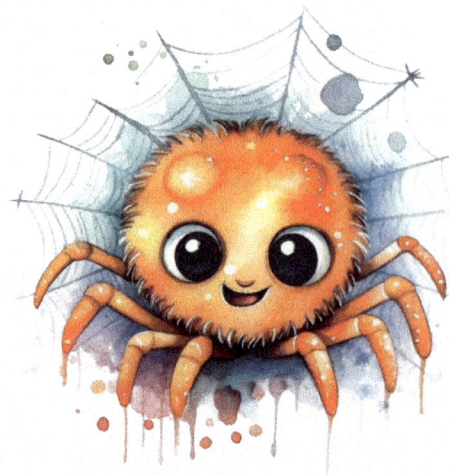

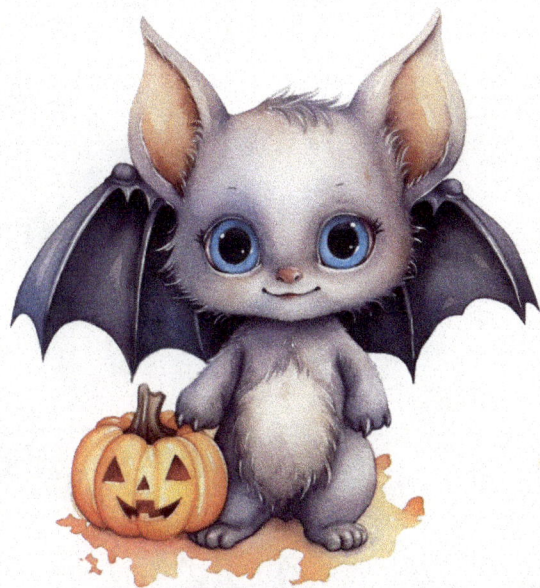

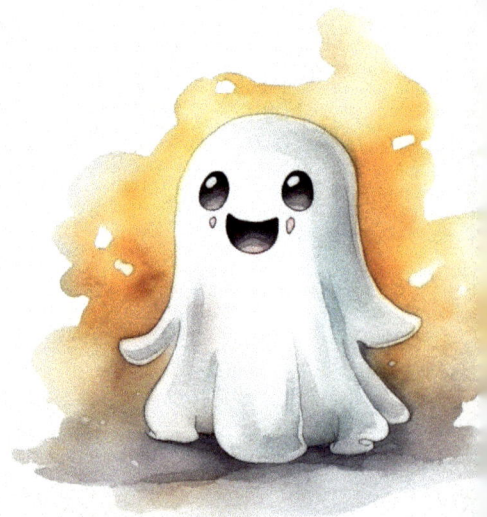

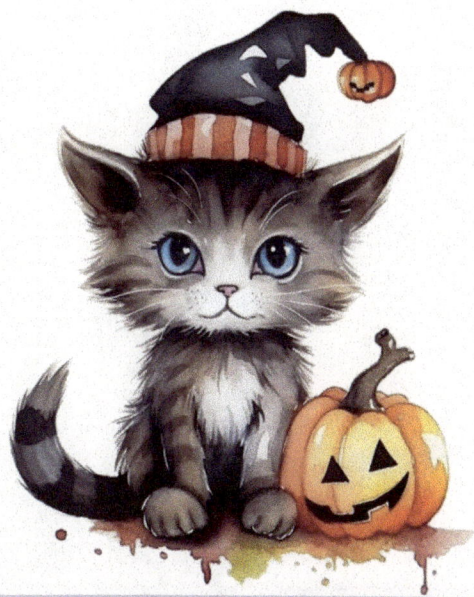

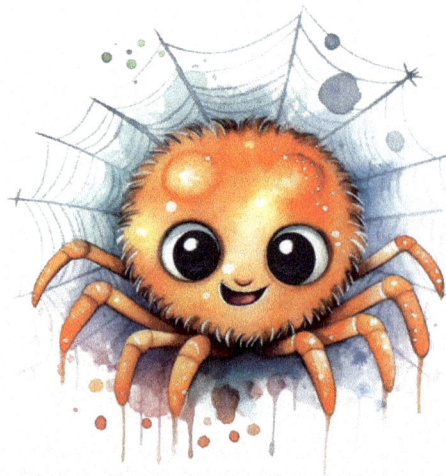

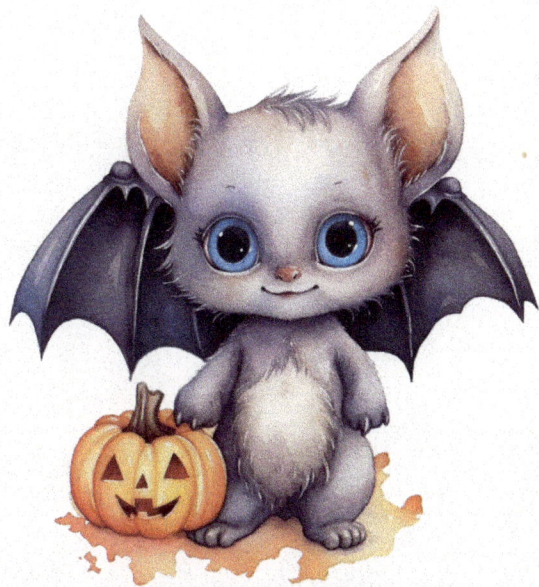

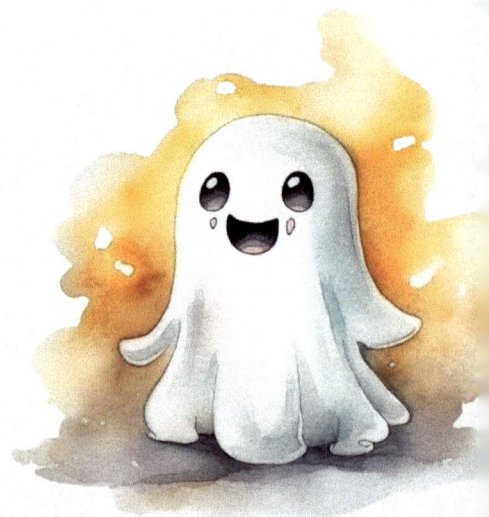

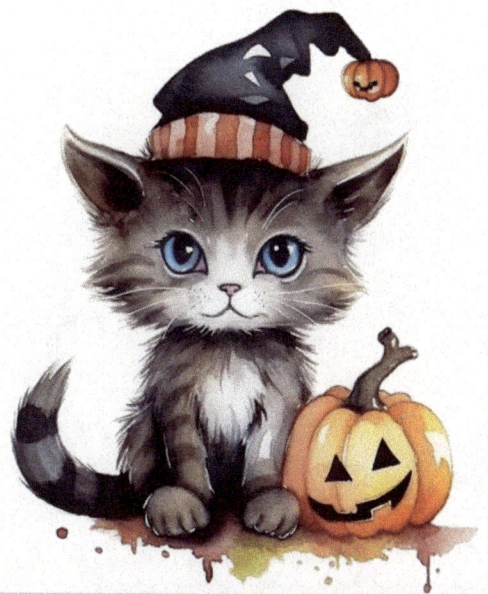

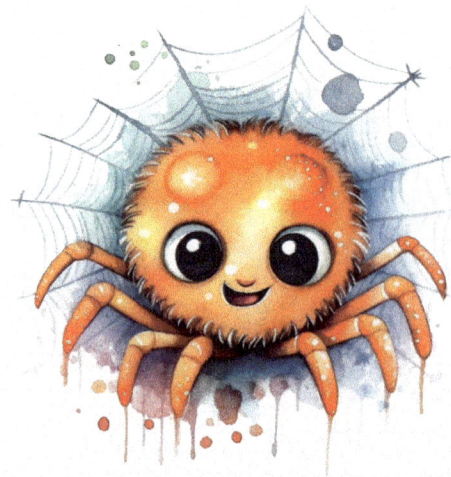

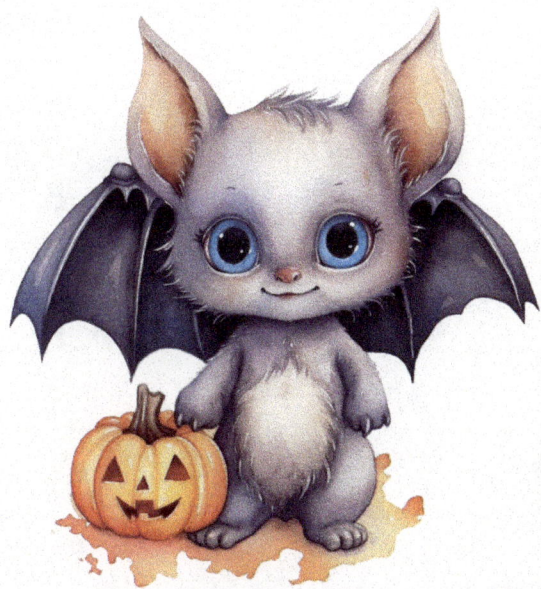

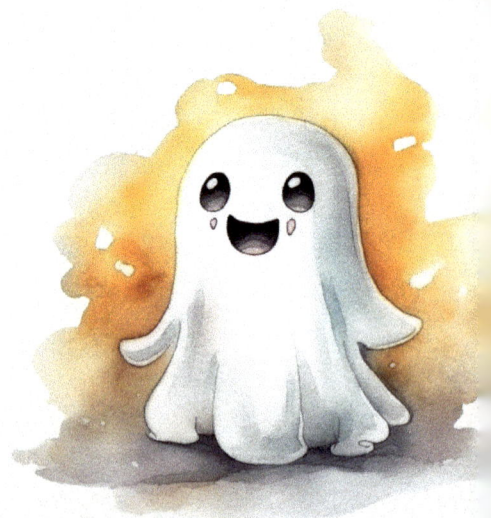

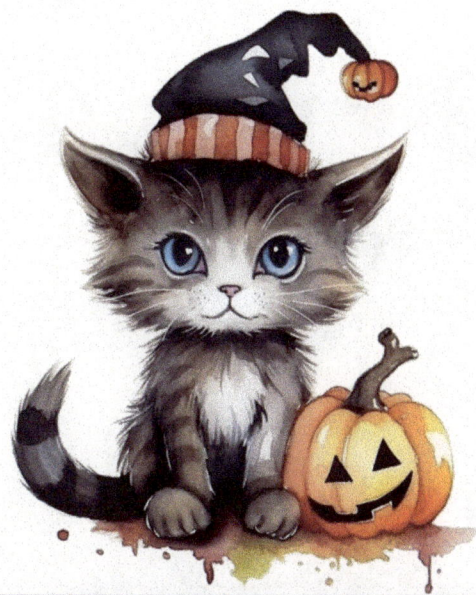

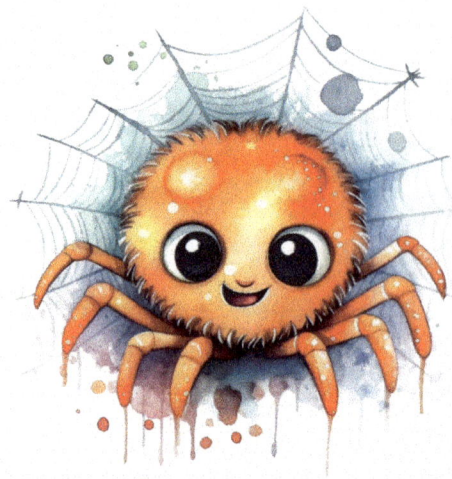

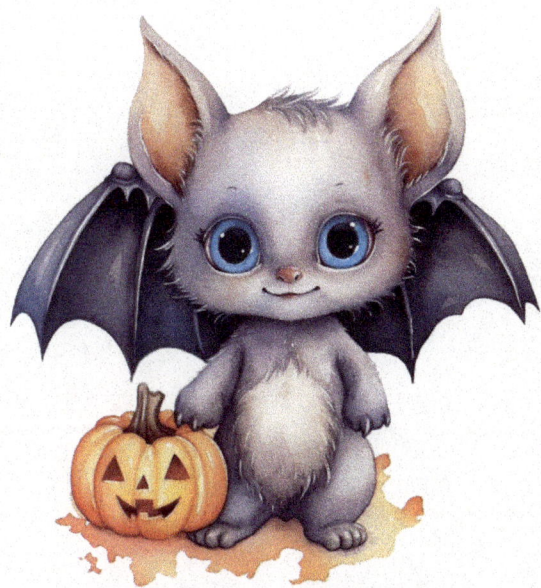

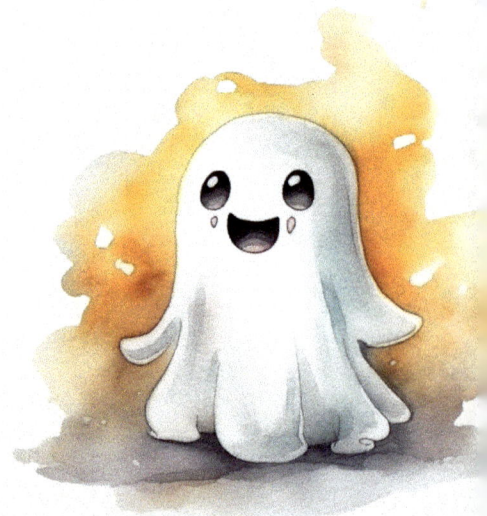

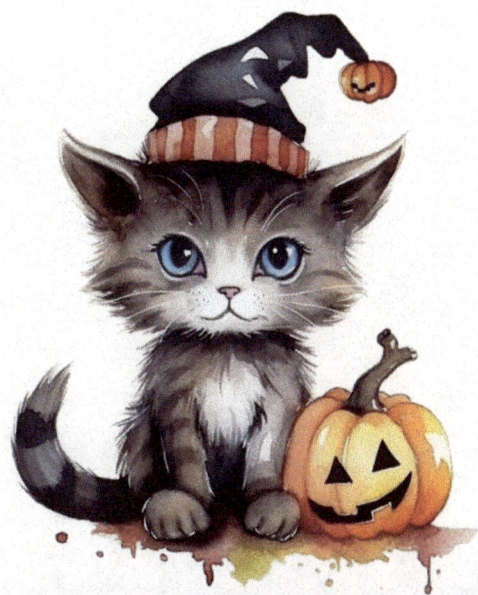

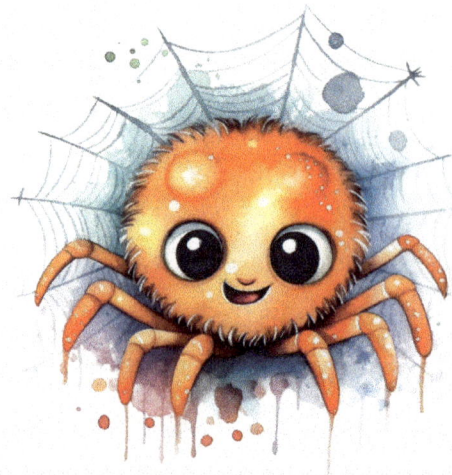

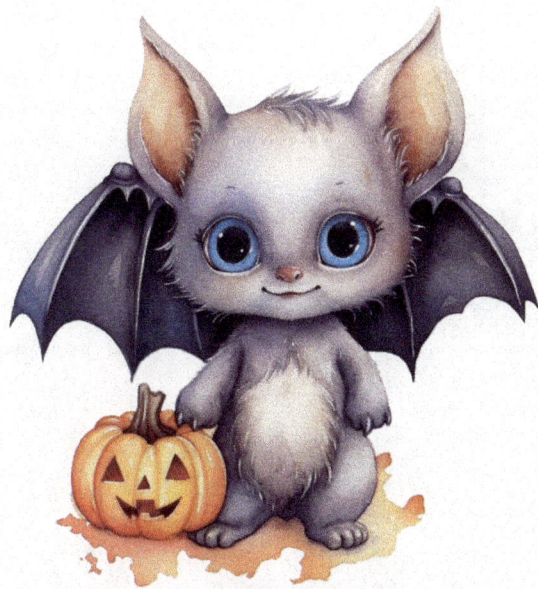

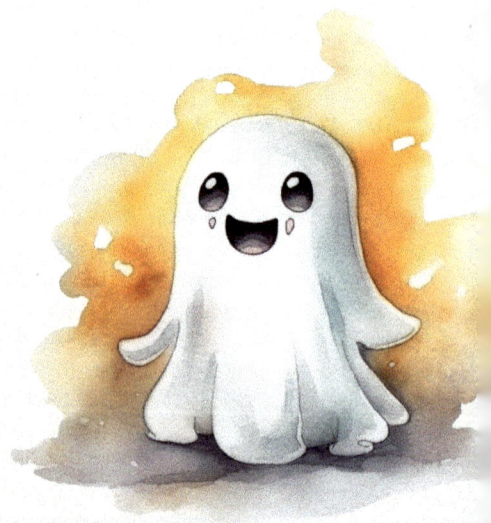

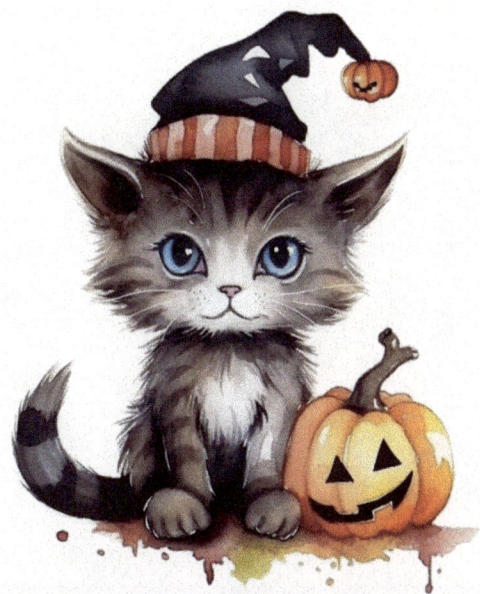

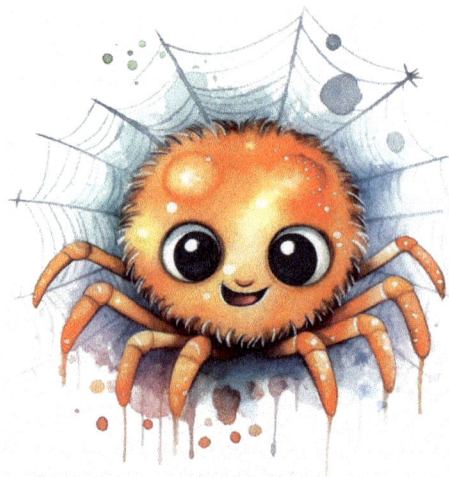

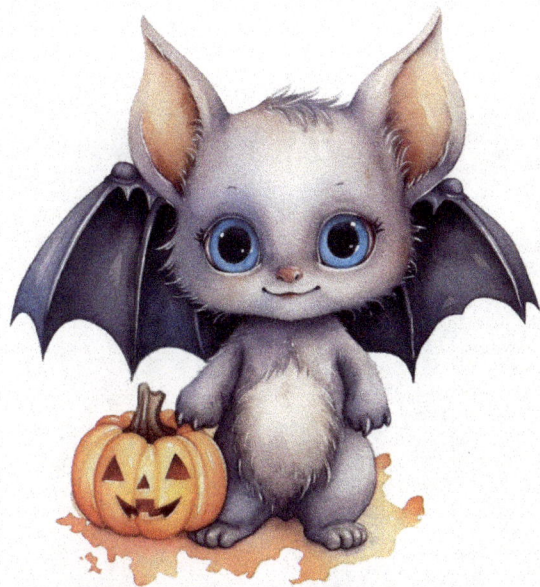

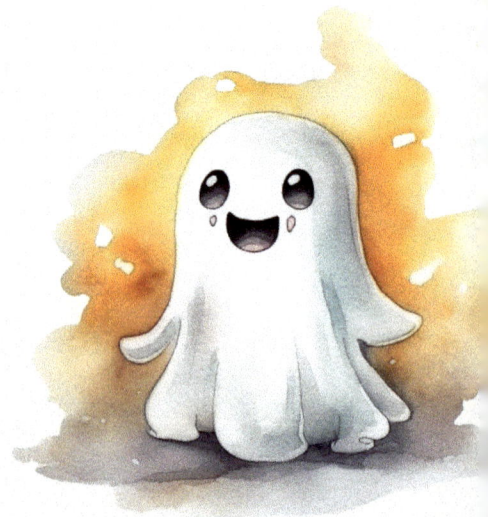

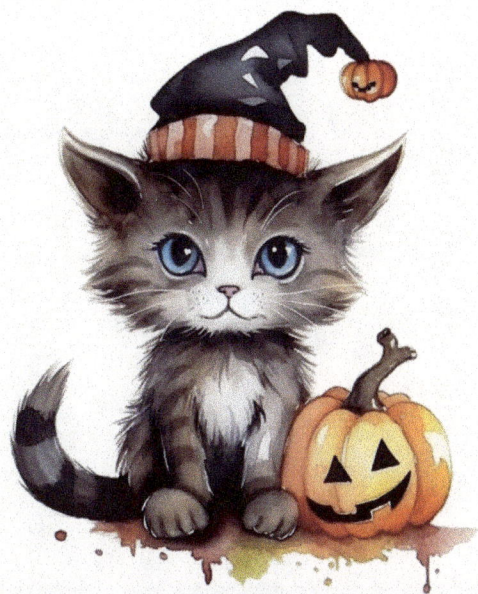

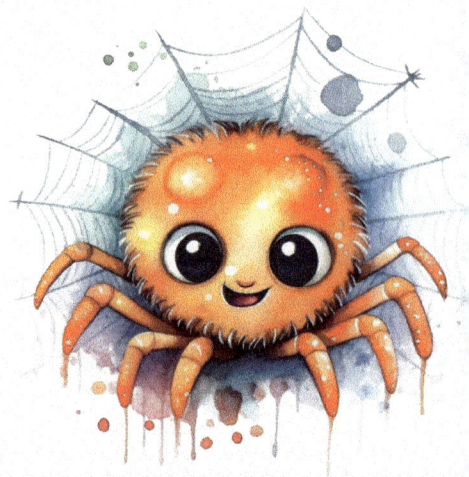

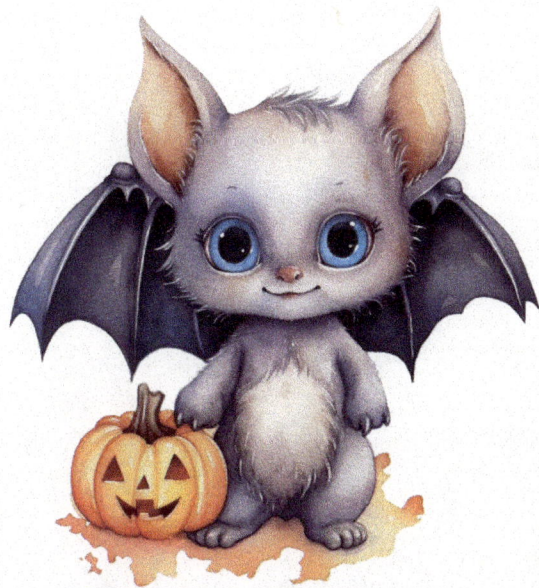

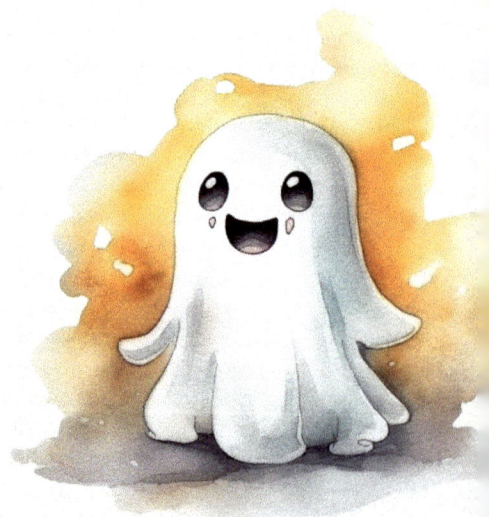

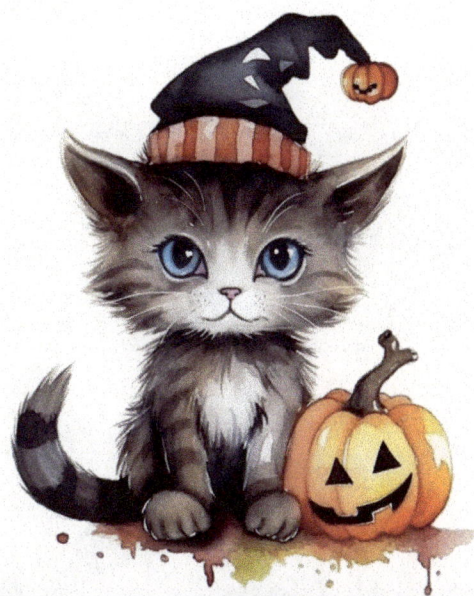

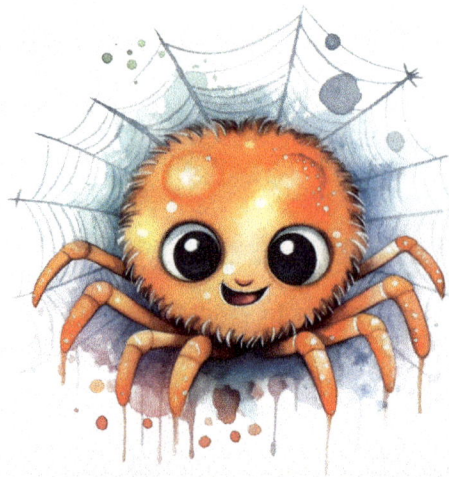

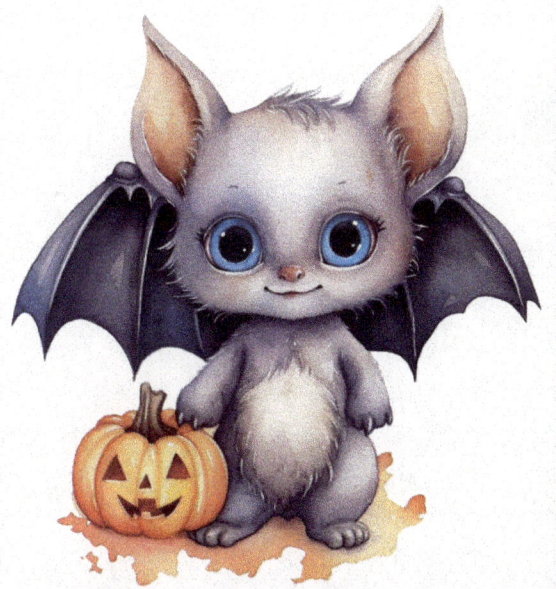

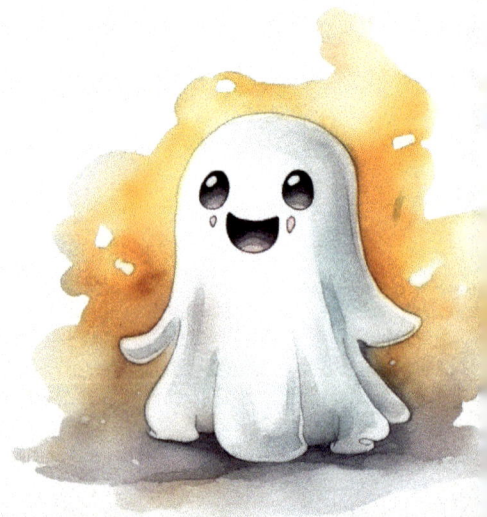

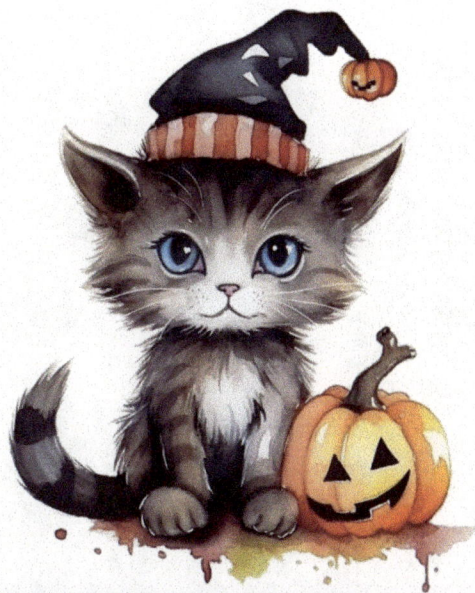

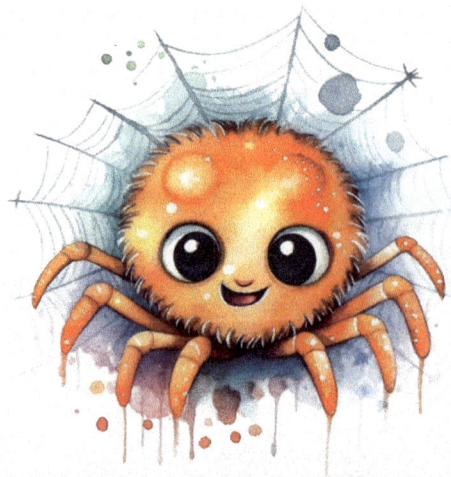

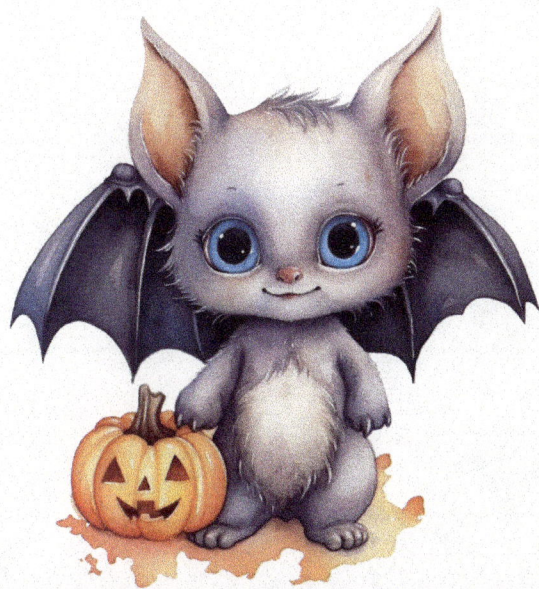

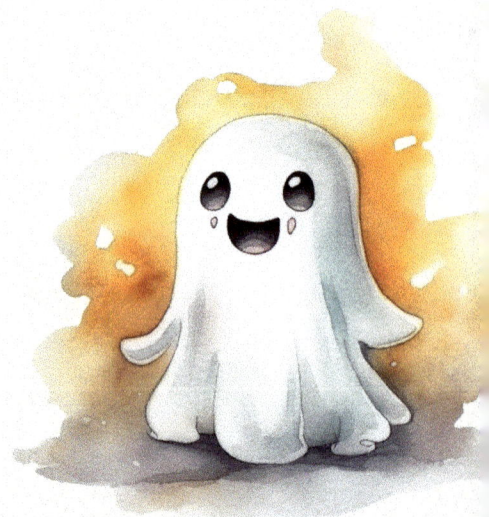

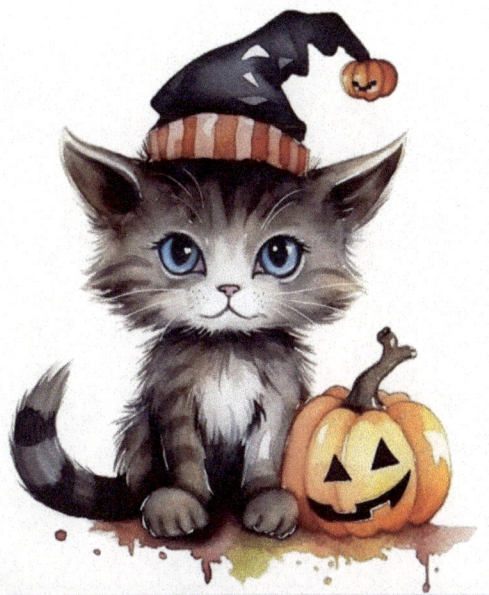

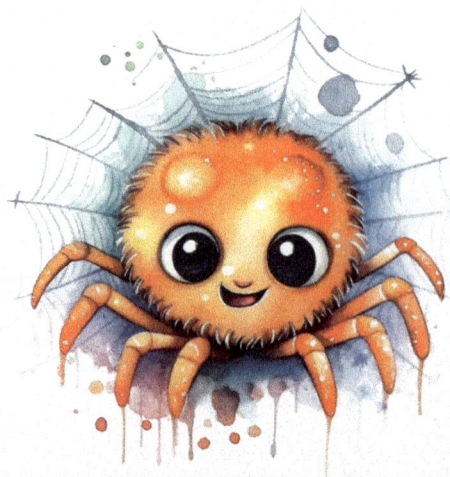

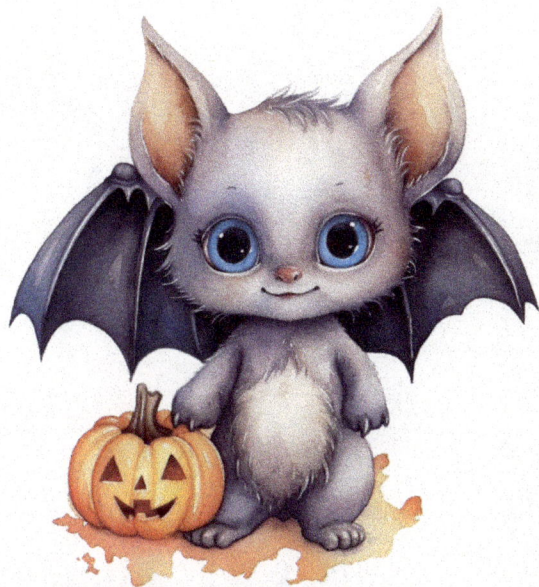

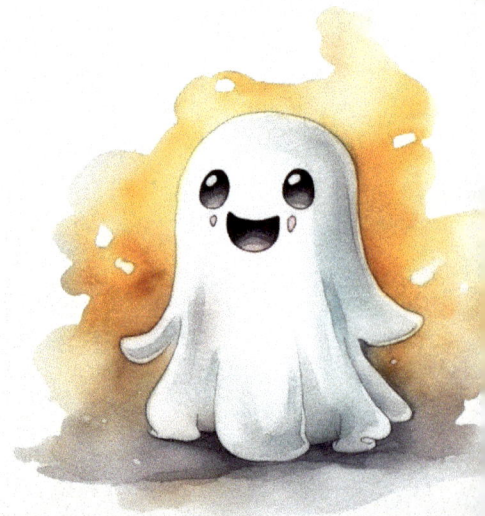

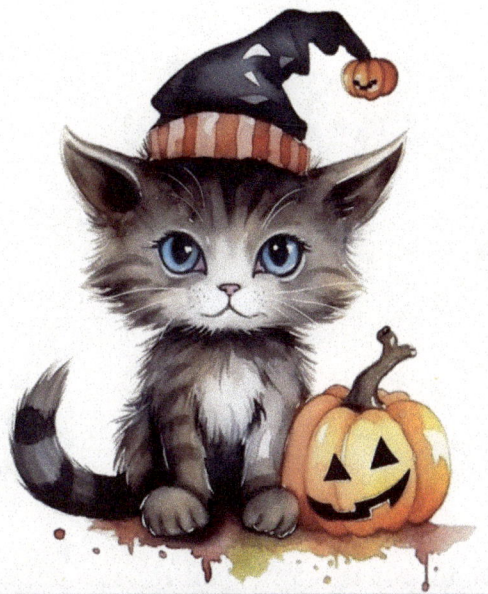

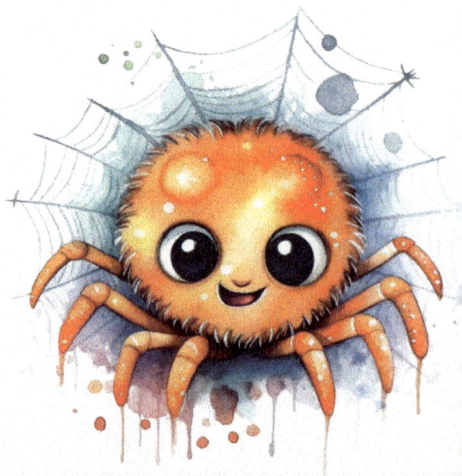

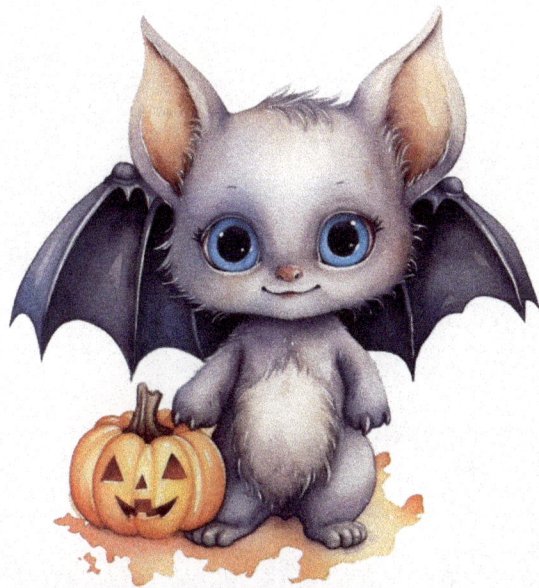

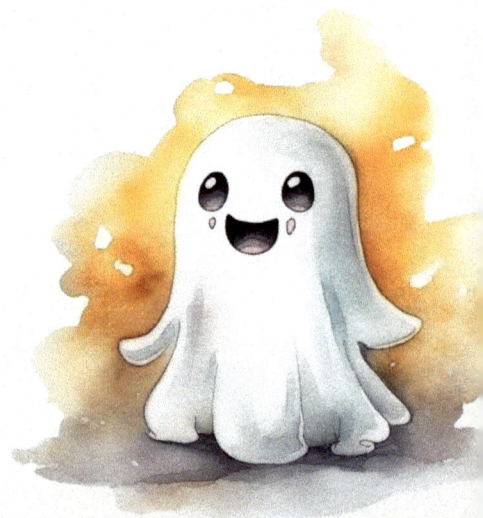

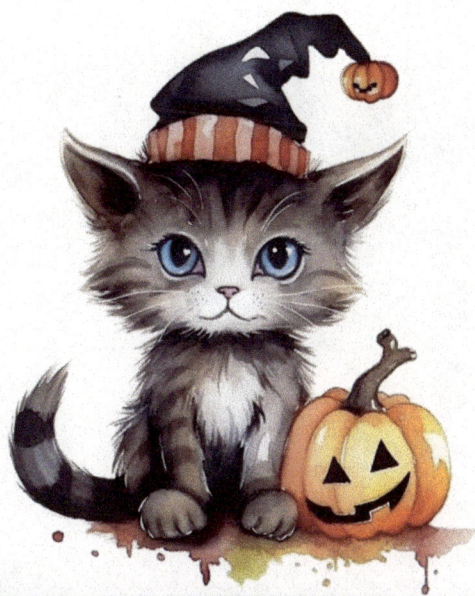

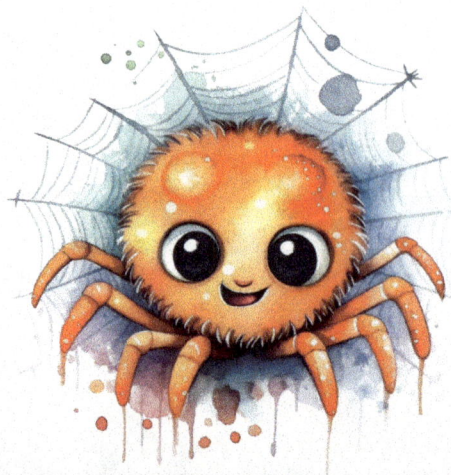

Name	Gift

Name	Gift

Name	Gift

Name	Gift

Name	Gift

Name	Gift

Name	Gift

Name	Gift

www.ingramcontent.com/pod-product-compliance
Lightning Source LLC
Chambersburg PA
CBHW061748260326
41914CB00006B/1029